The Ultimate Paleo Shopping Guide

All You Need For a Paleo Lifestyle

I0413269

Disclaimer

The ideas, concepts and opinions expressed in this book are intended to be used for educational purposes only. This book is provided with the understanding that authors and publisher are not rendering medical advice of any kind, nor is this book intended to replace medical advice, nor to diagnose, prescribe or treat any disease, condition, illness or injury.

It is imperative that before beginning any diet or exercise program, you receive full medical clearance from a licensed physician. Author and publisher claim no responsibility to any person or entity for any liability, loss, or damage caused or alleged to be caused directly or indirectly as a result of the use, application or interpretation of the material in this book.

Why Is This Book The Ultimate Paleo Book?

Paleo, or the lifestyle of the caveman, as it is better known, is a simpler and healthier way of eating. In this particular lifestyle, you should only consume the foods that were available at the time of our ancestors, the caveman. Hence, you cannot eat any item of food that was not available to them.

Further on in the book, we will not only discuss what Paleo is, but also the benefits you can gain by following this lifestyle. The sole purpose of this book is to share with you, the wide variety of foods you can eat on Paleo and of course the grey areas of Paleo as well.

Thus in this book you will find:

- Discussion on Paleo
- Benefits of Paleo
- Foods allowed on Paleo
- Shopping list of Paleo foods

Read on to find out more.

Table of Contents

Chapter 1- An Introduction to Paleo

"The foundation of success in life is good health, that is the substratum fortune; it is also the basis of happiness. A person cannot accumulate a fortune very well when he is sick."

-P. T. Barnum

"He, who has health, has hope.

And he, who has hope, has everything."

-Benjamin Franklin

What is the Paleo Diet?

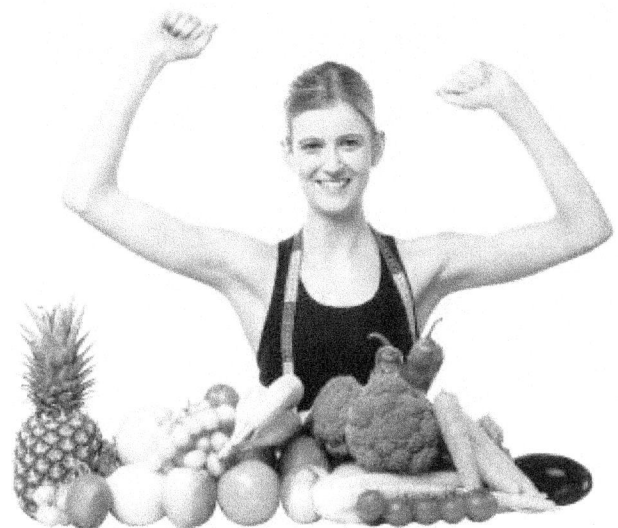

Simply put, the Paleo diet follows the lifestyle and eating habits of our ancestors, the caveman. Our ancestors were hunters and gatherers, who foraged and hunted for food. To them, food was only a source of energy and thus, required for their survival. Therefore, they ate what was available to them.

Similarly, the concept behind the Paleo diet is to eat as our ancestors ate. Well, not exactly as they did! No one expects us to hunt and gather food. Instead, the idea is to eat only those foods that were available to them.

Thus we eat only natural food, those that are provided to us by nature and none of the processed versions that although look like food, give us none of the nutrition or benefits that it should.

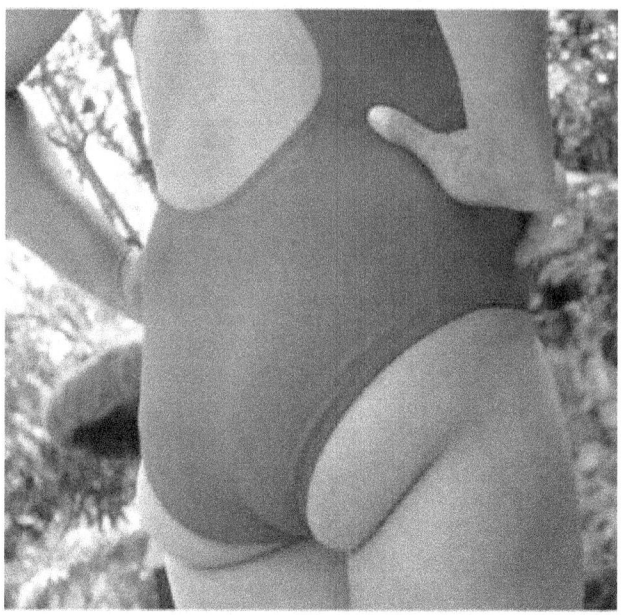

Instead of the processed food we consume, we were originally supposed to eat these natural foods such as fruits, vegetables, grains, fishes, chicken and other sources of meat. These foods contain within them, all the nutrition we need for optimal functioning of our body.

On the other hand, the processed food that most of us eat today, in one form or another, is the reason behind many of the diseases we suffer from.

Many cardiovascular diseases, diabetes, kidney, blood disorder, or any of the wide variety of disorders now commonly known to man, are solely due to the foods we consume.

Through research and studies, we are wiser to the lifestyles of our ancestors and also the fact that they didn't suffer from any of these diseases. The reason behind their health was their active lifestyle and the consumption of only natural food.

If we follow the same lifestyle, we could free ourselves from the affliction of modern lifestyle and become healthier and live happier lives. This has been proven to us by those, who have been following the Paleo lifestyle since for years and are not only happier, healthier but flourishing in every way possible.

Chapter 2- The Benefits of Paleo!

"Love is not as important as good health. You cannot be in love if you're not healthy. You can't appreciate it."

-Bryan Cranston

The Benefits of Paleo!

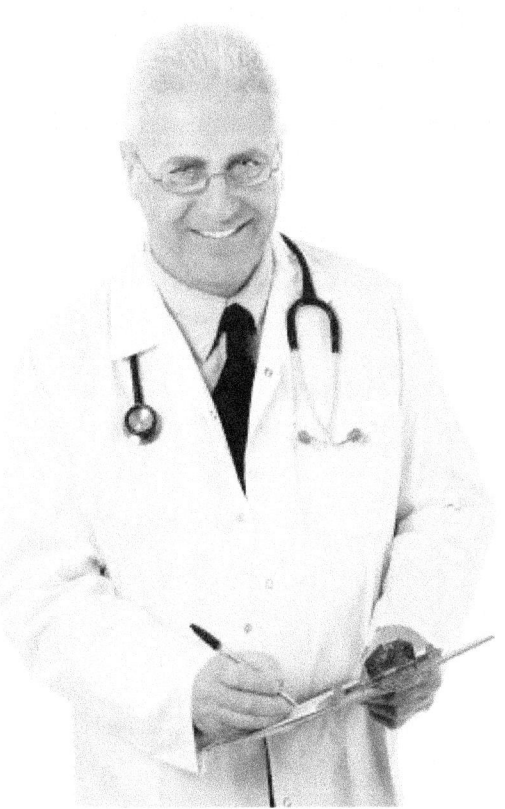

The struggle we go through every day is in the pursuit of happiness, in one way or other. Strangely enough, everyone believes, that happiness comes hand in hand with success and richness. Yet we can see that the rich people in this world are equally miserable!

Where does the key of** Happiness **lie then?

To be happy, it is essential that we remain healthy as well. A healthy mind, body and soul create a feeling of general wellbeing. Yet, we all neglect our health in return for success. If only we could focus on our health first and rest later, we could live truly enriched lives.

The first of the many benefits that are experienced by those following the Paleo diet is a feeling of contentment and happiness. Once a person starts eating all natural and minimally processed food, they start feeling good every day. As a result almost every day is a happy day.

No wonder the people following the Paleo lifestyle love it so much!

The second problem with most of us is that we feel lethargic all day! There are very few morning persons in the world. The rest of us, take till noon to truly wake up and start focusing on our tasks, only to get back in to a zombie state by mid-afternoon. We cannot wait to collapse on our beds and go to sleep, all the while, dreading going back to work the next day.

People following the Paleo lifestyle, claim to have more energy, throughout the day! They actually get a lot done in a day now, compared to their previous performance levels.

Many people claim that they feel, as if they had been half awake throughout their lives, until they started eating all natural, non-processed food.

It is very common to see people going through therapies, for one reason or another, throughout their lives. Anti-anxiety pills are selling like mints!

What has happened to us?

It feels as if we have stopped living; instead we are just going through the motions, day after day just for the sake of it.

This is again, amongst the first few changes that people on the caveman diet, notice about themselves. A feeling of being truly free, a peace of mind they had only experienced a rare few times in their lives.

They feel more focused, more alert, and less prone to jump at small annoyances.

Wishing you could get a massage? Or find some way to relieve the muscle soreness?

This is another one of the great benefits of eating like our ancestors, your body starts getting flexible, not very unlike the bodies of our ancestors who needed flexibility to hunt and chase animals every day.

Once you start eating according to the Paleo diet, you can say good-bye to the bloating and water retention, and say hello to long lean muscles and newfound flexibility.

Most of us have tried multiple diets and managed successfully to lose quite a few pounds, but unfortunately gained most of it back again! Similarly people on the Paleo diet, have experienced great weight loss and fat loss results as well, but this time the results are different.

These pounds, once gone, are not coming back, unless of course you start bingeing on processed food once again. Weight loss, is one of the most sought after benefits of the Paleo diet.

It is due to the low carb nature of this diet that pounds fall off of you with incredible ease.

Hair fall, skin problems and common diseases we suffer from, add ten or so years to our faces, making us look older than we actually are. Like most people, followers of the Paleo diet also tried one miracle cream, after another and became more and more disappointed after each attempt.

These people saw great transformations in their skin and faces, after they had been on Paleo for a few weeks. They felt their skin look younger, start glowing and their skin problems disappeared gradually too.

The true miracle in this diet is only till the extent of the miracle that resides in nature. No miracle cream can contain the benefits one can avail from consuming natural food that is packed with nutrition, while eliminating 'toxic' food completely.

Even though many of us, long for our beds throughout the day, amazingly none of us feel any better after we wake up from a long night's sleep. Isn't that very confusing?

No matter how long we sleep for, we never feel energized!

On the other hand, the people following the caveman diet, not only feel energized throughout the day, they also sleep better and wake up refreshed!

Chapter 3- Foods Allowed on Paleo!

"A man's health can be judged by which he takes two at a time - pills or stairs."

-Joan Welsh

"You are, what you eat"

-Victor Lindlahr

Foods Allowed on Paleo!

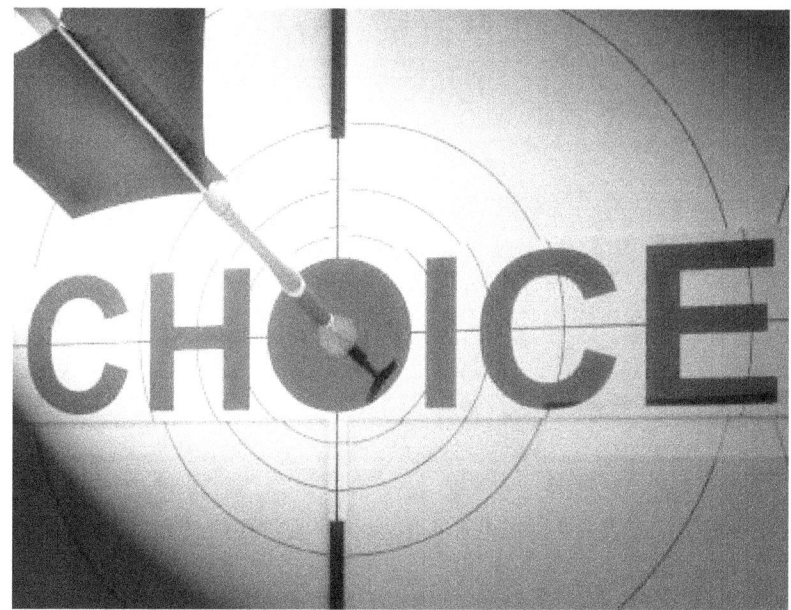

Basic Principles

The basic rules of Paleo are very simple. Even though there are many arguments surrounding

Paleo, these basic principals remain the same.

- Make protein a priority in every meal. Your protein should come from a variety of meat including, seafood, and eggs.

- Include moderate amounts of good fats in every meal such as starchy vegetables, fruits, and nuts.

- Keep the amount of grains such as corn, rice, legumes, and wheat to a minimum.

- Drink a lot of water and green tea.

Tips

Although you should always keep to the basic principles of Paleo diet, these are some additional tips that will help you make the most out of it.

Purchase the best quality food that is available in the market and invest in organic food whenever you can. To better understand what type of food to purchase, here are some food preference tips.

- Purchase local food whenever you have a lot of food options at hand.

- Always purchase organic when available.

- Choose grass-fed meats and animal protein.

- Do not eat meat from animals that have been caged.

- Eat only unpasteurized dairy which is not processed.

- Choose natural clean produce that is pesticides and hormone free.

Fruits and Vegetables

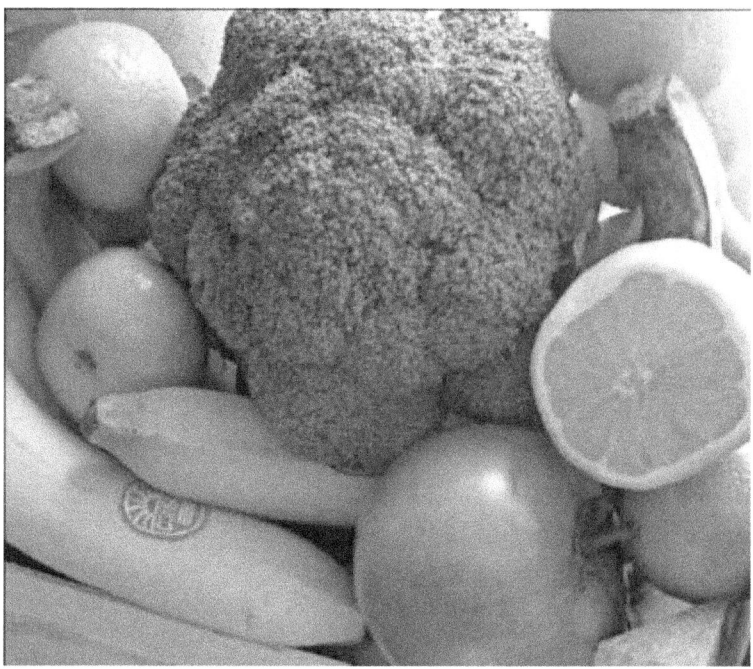

The sole purpose of the Paleo diet is to eat clean, natural food. The food available in the market is filled with pesticides, making these foods harmful for you, as a result. It is best to choose organic fruits and vegetables whenever you can.

Even though expensive, they will save you from heavy medical bills in the long run. These chemicals severely mess up our bodies, and hence become the reason behind many of our illnesses. In short, opt for organic fruits and vegetables or grow your own produce. It will save you expenses in the long run.

- Eat a lot of vegetables and fruits.

- Buy the fruits and vegetables that are in season and freeze them for later use. This will not only make them more affordable but also keep the nutrition content intact.

- Stock up on fruits and vegetables that are on sale.

- Choose a lot of leafy vegetables and colorful fruits.

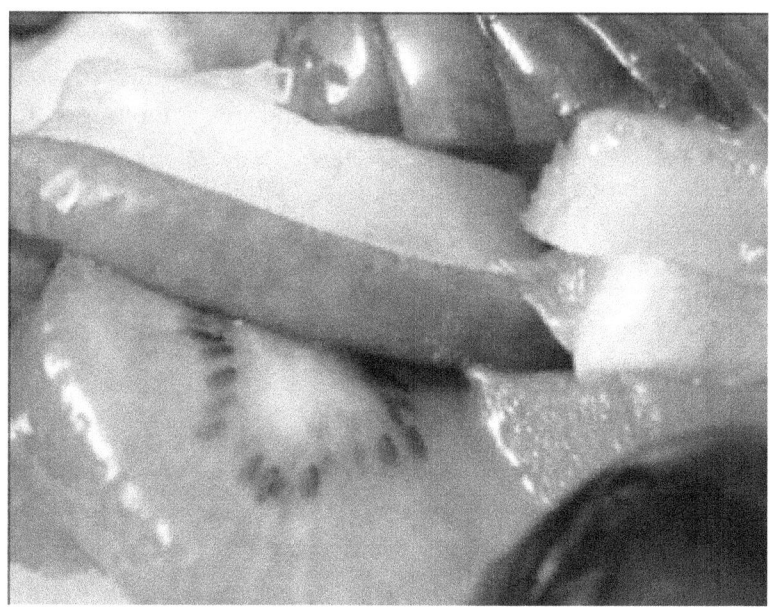

- Plums

- Cantaloupe

- Apple

- Avocado

- Banana

- Passion Fruit

- Lime

- Blueberries

- Boysenberries

- Cherries

- Cranberries

- Figs

- Grapefruit

- Guava

- Honeydew melon

- Lemon

- Blackberries

- Mango

- Orange

- Papaya

- Peaches

- Pears

- Gooseberries

- Lychee

- Pineapple

- Pomegranate

- Rhubarb

- Grapes

- Star Fruit

- Kiwi

- Raspberries

- Strawberries

- Tangerine

- Watermelon

- Apricot

Vegetables Allowed on Paleo

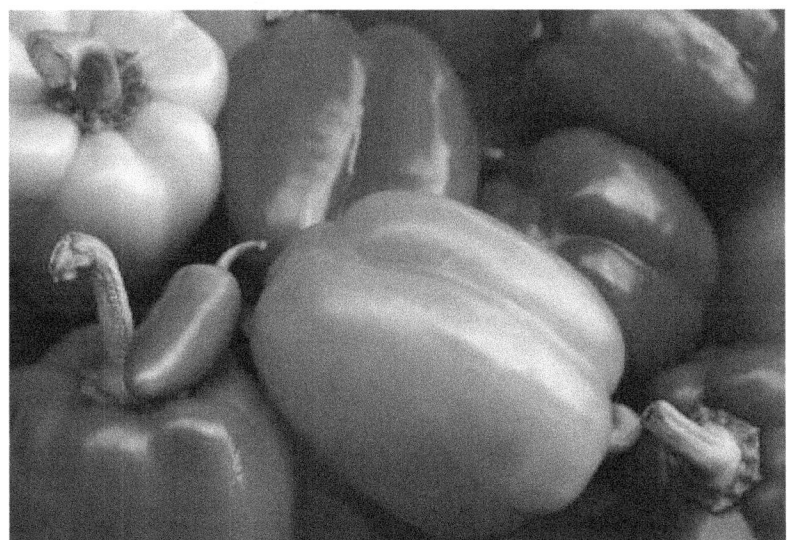

- Kohlrabi

- Bell Peppers

- Mustard Greens

- Artichoke

- Beet Greens

- Squash

- Beets

- Broccoli

- Cabbage

- Celery

- Parsnip

- Cucumber

- Brussels Sprouts

- Dandelion

- Eggplant

- Green Onions

- Kale

- Collards

- Mushrooms

- Onions

- Cauliflower

- Parsley

- Peppers

- Pumpkin

- Radish

- Carrots

- Seaweed

- Spinach

- Swiss Chard

- Tomato

- Turnip Greens

- Turnips

- Watercress

- Lettuce

- Asparagus

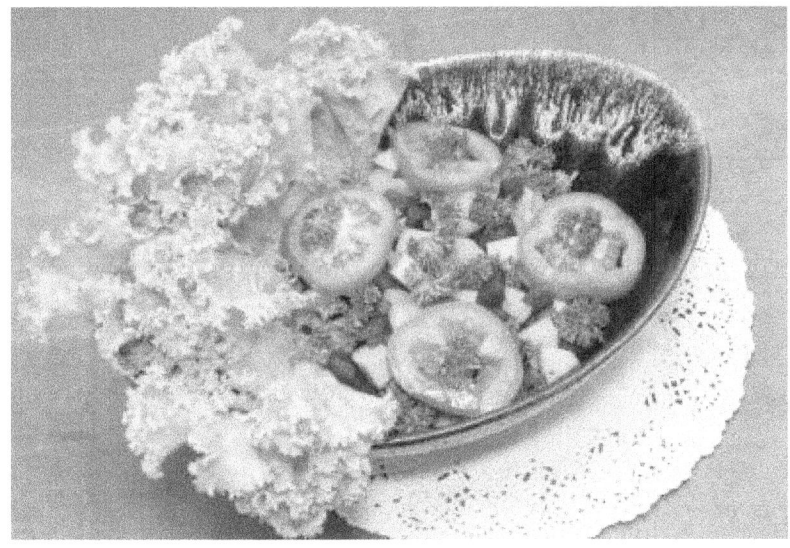

Meat

Similar to the issue with vegetables and fruits, the meat available these days, is so contaminated and chemical-laden, that it is hardly safe to. The hormones and antibiotic filled meat that we consume on a regular basis, leads to diseases instead of making us any healthier.

Thus it is crucial to understand which meat is safe for consumption.

- Always choose organic and grass-fed meat whenever available. This is the safest and healthiest meat available.

- If organic and grass-fed meat is unavailable, lean meat is the next best option.

- In fish, choose wild caught or catch them yourself whenever possible.

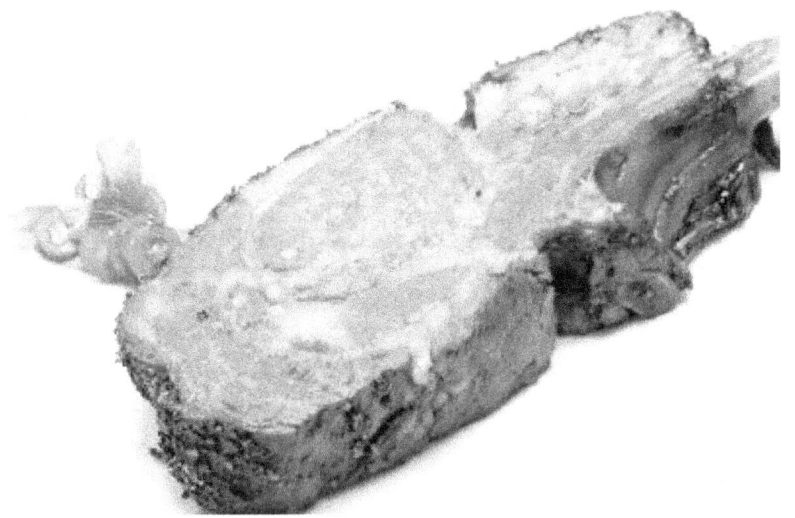

- Flank Steak

- Chicken livers

- Chicken

- Chicken breast

- Chuck Steak

- Pork Chops

- Duck

- Eggs

- Extra lean hamburger

- Goat meat

- Goose

- Lean Beef Trimmed

- Lean poultry

- Lean veal

- Organ meats of Beef, lamb, pork

- Pork loin

- Rabbit meat

- Top Sirloin Steak

- Turkey breast

- Lean Pork Trimmed

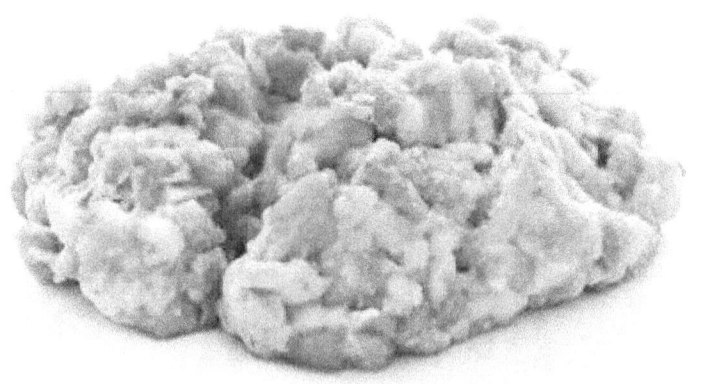

Fish Allowed on Paleo

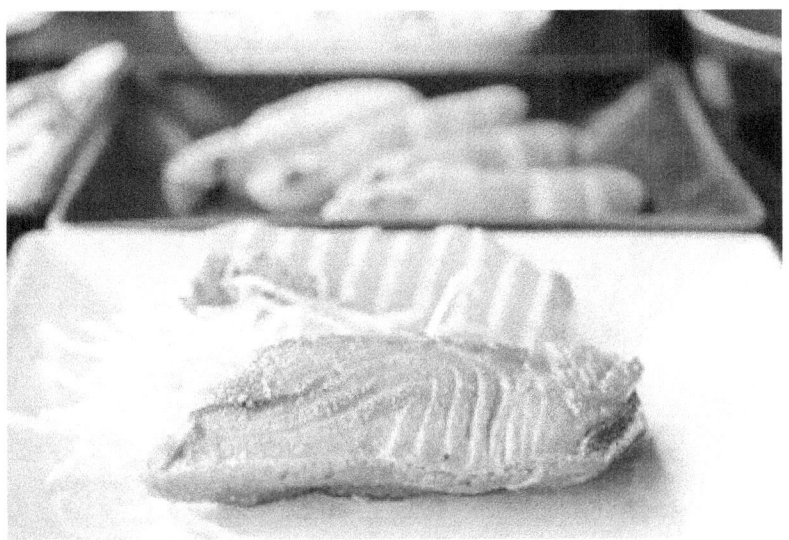

- Striped bass

- Bass

- Cod

- Eel

- Flatfish

- Turbot

- Grouper

- Haddock

- Halibut

- Herring

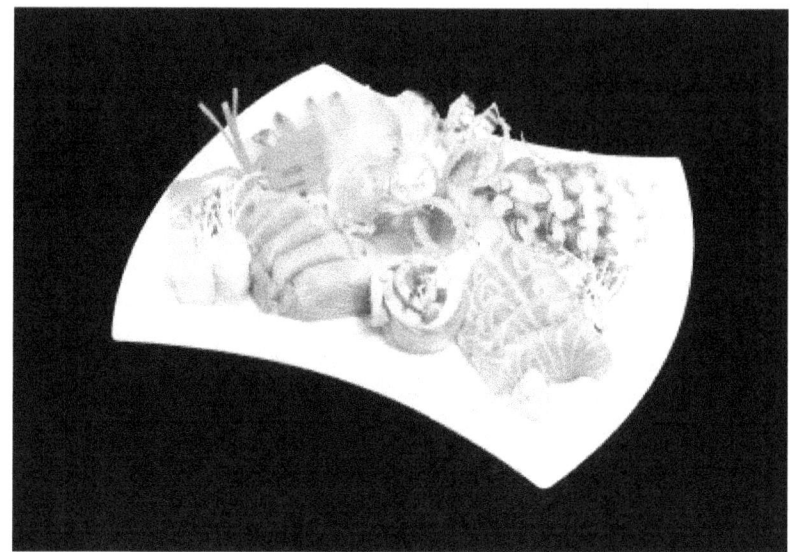

- Mackerel

- Mullet

- Perch

- Pike

- Red snapper

- Salmon

- Scrod

- Shark

- Sunfish

- Tilapia

- Drum

- Trout

- Tuna

- Rockfish

Shellfish Allowed on Paleo

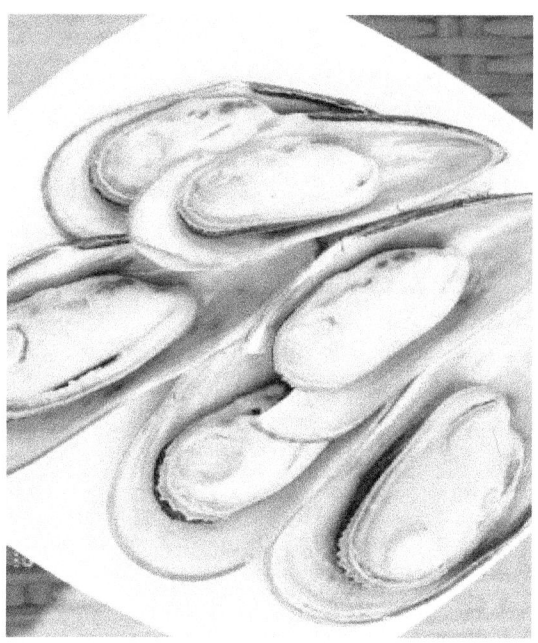

- Lobster

- Mussels

- Crab

- Clams

- Crayfish

- Scallops

- Oysters

- Shrimp

Fats

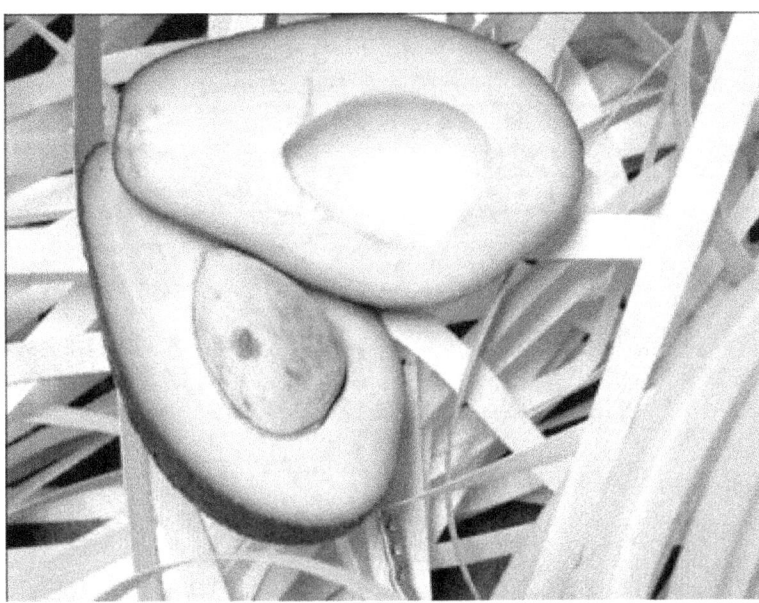

As per popular myths, fat is a forbidden food. Well, as per researches and studies, fat is of two types, there are good fats and bad fats.

Why is Fat Important?

Healthy Fat is essential for cell formation and proper function of our system. If instead of healthy fats, we continue to eat unhealthy or bad quality fats, we will find ourselves facing many health problems. Poor quality fats and oils lead to poor quality cells and subsequent health problems.

Nuts, Seeds and Fats Allowed on Paleo

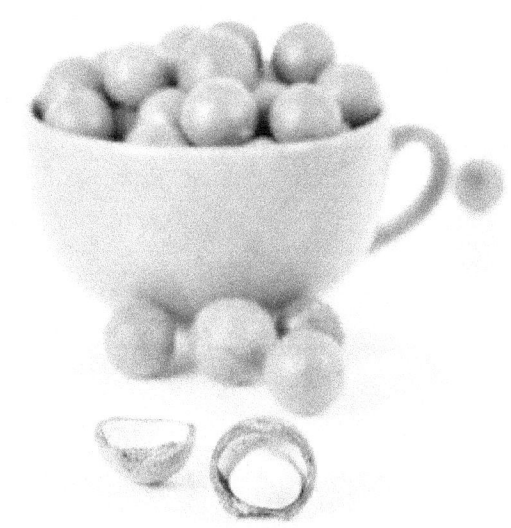

- Macadamia Nuts

- Almonds

- Almond Butter

- Pine Nuts

- Pistachios (unsalted)

- Cashews

- Sunflower Seeds

- Sesame Seeds

- Brazil Nuts

- Pumpkin Seeds

- Hazelnuts

- Pecans

Chapter 4: Food Items Allowed In Moderation in Paleo

"The best and most efficient pharmacy is within your own system."

-Robert C. Peale

"Let food be thy medicine and medicine be thy food"

— Hippocrates

Food Items Allowed In Moderation in Paleo

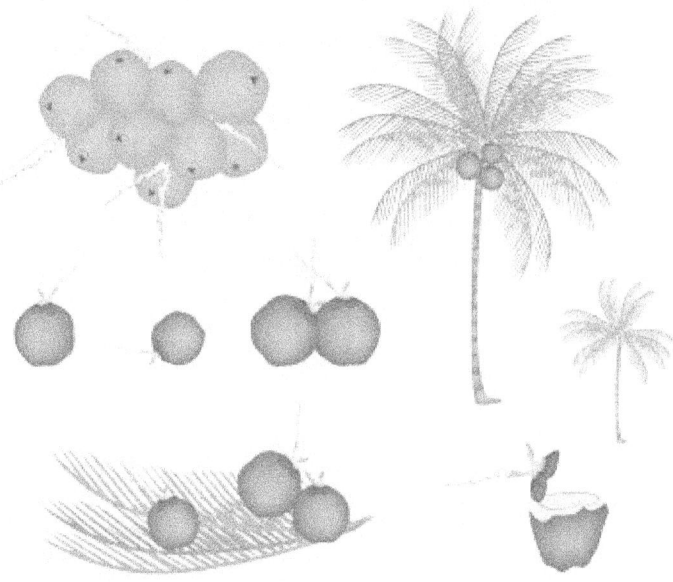

Even though these food items are allowed in Paleo, they should be eaten in moderation, as too much of any of these food items, is not good for health. The sole purpose of Paleo is to get healthy and avail all the benefits that come with being healthy.

For that purpose, it is essential to consume these food items in moderation otherwise the purpose of Paleo would be lost. The importance of this point increases manifolds for those who are following Paleo to lose weight. So, it is not only important that you eat healthy, it is also crucial that you eat smart.

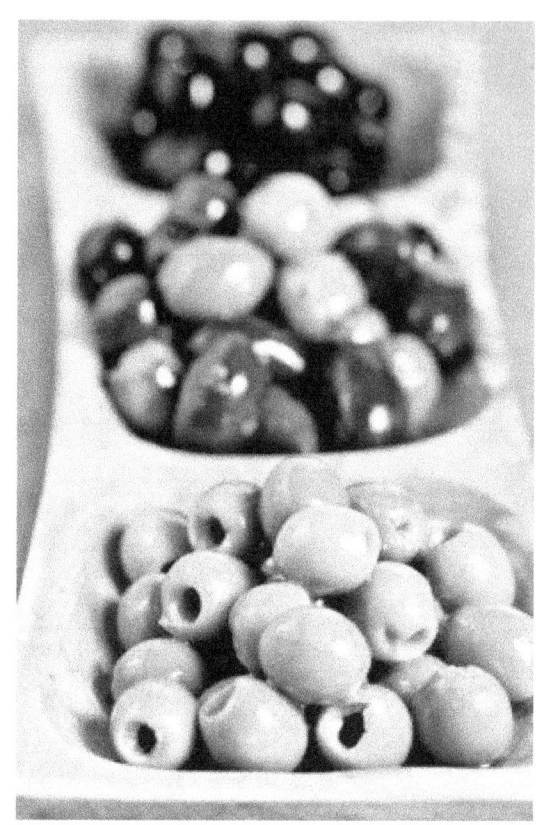

- Coffee

- Canola Oils

- Olive

- Diet Sodas

- Walnut

- Flaxseed

- Tea

- Avocado

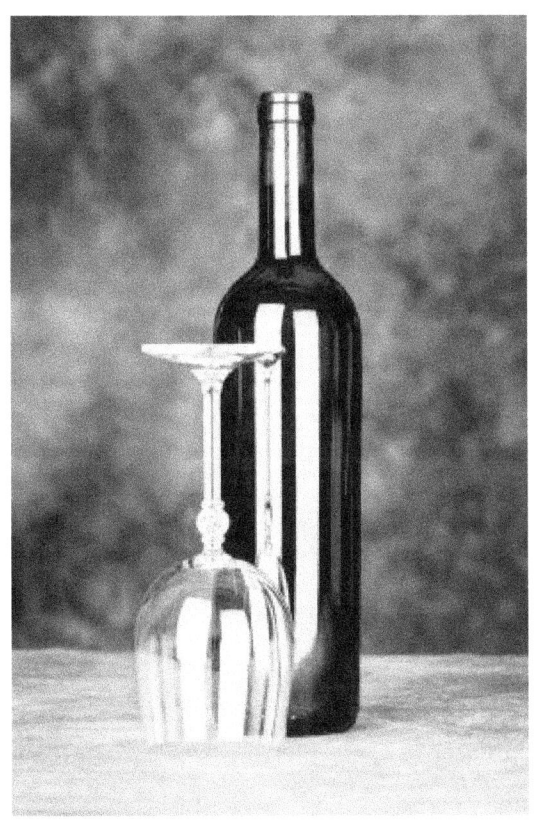

- Honey

- Wine

- Spirits

- Beer

- Dark Chocolate

- Almond Flour

- Coconut Flour

Ready to Shop?

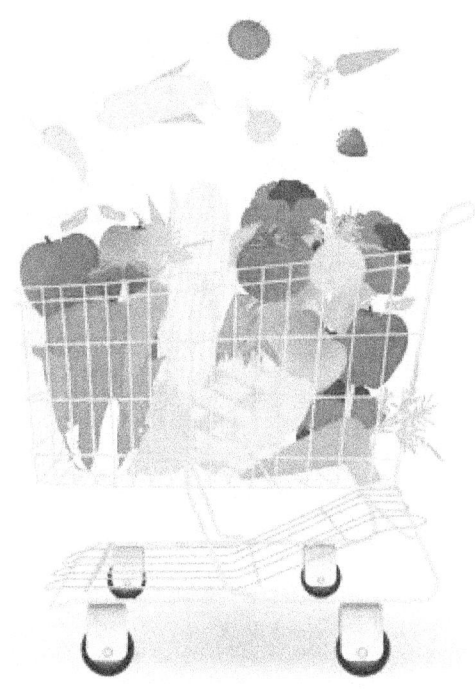

Now that you are fully equipped with a comprehensive shopping list, comprising of all the Paleo food items you will need, are you ready to shop your way to a healthier you?